POSITIVE THINKING
37 KEYS TO MAXIMIZING
YOUR LIFE

AFFIRMATIONS, MOTIVATION AND ACHIEVING

SUCCESS

About the Author

Dr. William E. Ackerman III is currently the Medical Director and CEO of the Pain Medicine Consultants Group, PA in Little Rock and Conway, Arkansas. He is a Board certified anesthesiologist and completed a fellowship in pain medicine and currently practices pain management. Dr. Ackerman is furthermore, board certified in pain medicine. He has been a Lt. Col. and Chief of Anesthesiology at two Army medical centers. He has had an extensive successful academic career and is now in private practice. He also has been an Associate Professor and Director of an academic pain center. He has been on the academy faculty at three medical schools. He has published over 135 scientific articles in peer reviewed journals. He has published and presented scientific abstracts at international and national academic meetings. He has lectured at medical schools and various scientific meetings. Dr. Ackerman has published many chapters in academic textbooks as well. He has published nine books. He has been on the Editorial Board of two peer reviewed medical journals. He was nominated previously for the Southern Medical Society Medical Research Award and the Bristol-Meyers Squibb award for distinguished achievement in Pain Research. He was the recipient of the Karl Koeller research grant from the American Society of Regional Anesthesia and Pain Medicine. He has a strong interest in diversity and appropriate pain management in different gender and ethnic groups. He does not believe that a "one size fits all" approach is medically appropriate. He was selected previously to "Who's Who in International Medicine".

FREE BONUS: "CLICK THE LINK BELOW TO RECEIVE YOUR FREE EBOOKS!"

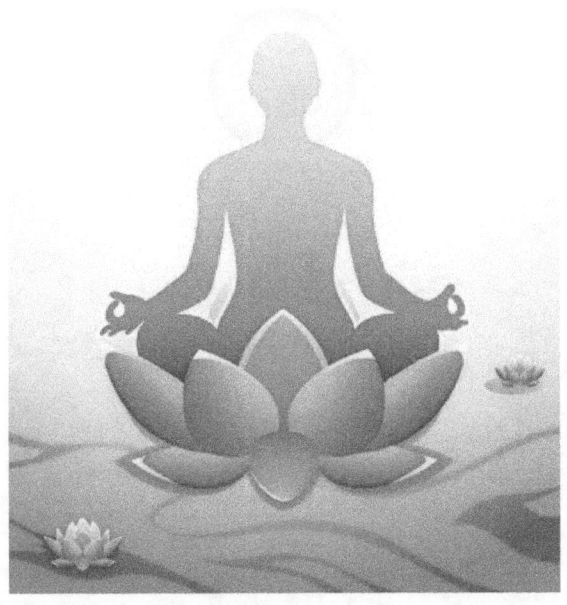

FREE BONUS "CLAIM YOUR FREE EBOOKS" BELOW FOR YOUR BONUS:

https://success321.leadpages.co/freebodymindsoul/

TABLE OF CONTENTS

INTRODUCTION

Have you ever wondered how positive thinking affects the outcome of your life? Life coaches know that it is the way forward to achieving your wildest dreams. You see these people telling you to discover your authentic self but they won't let you know how to use positive thinking to do that without charging you a fortune. However, if you could unlock the secrets, you could, in fact, plan the course of your life to such an extent that you actually achieve what your dreams tell you are the main aims that you have. Positive thinking is a very powerful tool to have on your side. In fact, those who are positive thinkers are always coming up in the newspapers all of the time and you may think of names such as Richard Branson, Bill Gates and Steve Jobs as being the epitome of success. They got to where they wanted to be because of their positive thinking and their belief in what they were doing. Inside of every person is this positive belief in something and it's time that you unleashed your positivity to make your world a better place to be.

This book gives you 37 pointers toward unlocking those secrets. Why? Because the actual route to doing this is more common sense than you may have imagined. There was a time when I believed that I could unlock those secrets and now that I have, it seems the right thing to do to pass these pointers on to you, so that you too can fulfill your dreams. Affirmations are only a small part of the picture. You need positive thinking and the right attitude if you want to unlock your own potential. You also need to work toward your goals and know that they are doable. If your belief is such that you can go toward your goals unflinchingly, you are more likely to reach them. In fact, many people don't know the direction their lives are heading in and leave much of what happens to them to chance. You only get one shot at it, so chance should never come into the picture.

Your success doesn't depend upon the good will of anyone else. Each of us has the same potential and that's the wonderful thing about the power of positive thinking. It allows you to find out what really makes you happy and set a course to achieve it. So what's the deal with positive thinking? Well, I can tell you from experience that it's more than just smiling and being happy. It's about using your positive attitude to learn all of the things you need to know in order to succeed and reach your goals, whether these are personal goals, financial goals or business goals. It doesn't matter what your dream is or how complex it appears to be, nor how simple. People don't all want the same things and it's your authenticity that will tell you what your dream is. Don't be swayed by anyone because it's YOUR dream not theirs. All I can do is point you in the right direction, so that you are more likely to achieve those goals.

There are thousands of people who go through life and who are dissatisfied with their lot in life. Why? Well, the reason is pretty clear when you study the individuals involved. They want more than they have but without actually being able to pinpoint what it is that they want, all they can do is criticize those who have elements of their dreams and put it down to good fortune. If they were to change their way of thinking and put a real label on what it is that they want, then they would bring all of these desires into the realms of possibility. That's when the magic starts to happen. This book goes through the process of explaining how positive thinking and motivation can work hand in hand to help you to succeed and to be happy at the same time.

Sometimes it takes the simplicity of childhood to actually live your dreams. Look a child whose dream it is to play a certain role in the pageant. Only one person will play that role and it won't always be the prettiest girl or the most handsome looking boy. Often it will be the child who showed that it was his/her dream to take that role and make the most of it that persuaded the teacher to let him/her have that role. When you grow up, what happens is that you are suddenly faced by complexity. Life isn't that simple any more. There are so many choices but there are also so many people in competition for different elements of life – The best car, the best house, the best wife, the best reputation – that people get confused about where they should be aiming. They begin to measure themselves against others and that's when dissatisfaction sets in. In fact, our world today encourages this kind of behavior by typecasting people, when in fact that may not be a fair representation of who a particular individual is.

When you learn to use positive thinking, you show the world the side of you that cannot be type-casted. You may call Bill Gates or Richard Branson entrepreneurial types, but you would never mistake one for the other because their style of entrepreneurship is so different. When you decide where you are going, you step out of the typecast and become a very strong individual with an awful lot to look forward to. Let's forget all of the pre-conditioning that you went through as a child. Today is the beginning of the rest of your life. Today matters and who you are today makes a difference to your future and your tomorrow.

CHAPTER ONE

UNLOCKING THE MYSTERY BEHIND NEGATIVE THOUGHT PROCESSES

Scientists and medical staff have long since recognized that there is a huge difference between people who have a negative outlook and those that have a positive outlook. It's almost like the difference between someone who sees the cup as half full compared with someone who sees the cup as half empty. The negative person will be the one that doesn't get what he wants in life because his negative attitude will always hold him back. You can even take this further if you need more explanation. If you were to put 20 individuals on a medical trial, supposing two people were given a placebo. Those two people may believe that they will get better and may very well improve in health because of their belief in the drug that they have taken. Medical placebos are well known and these work because there are no negative thought processes behind their use. Those that believe that they will work will experience great results. Such is the power of the mind. Conversely, you will have those that have no belief in the drug and perhaps they have a very negative mindset. These are the people who will always see the negative side of any situation. For them, it doesn't matter if the drug is real or placebo, it's their attitude that will decide the outcome.

Negative thought processes destroy people. They take away belief and they make the individual unhappy, stressed or even sick because of circumstance rather than illness itself. Achievement becomes a chore. People with a negative mindset are suspicious. They suspect other people's motives and they always find a reason why others succeed and they fail and it certainly won't be because of them. If you can imagine people looking out of the window at the world. Some will always see the skies as being blue and even when they are not, they will have hope that the sun will come through the clouds later. Negative people walk through their lives with a permanent cloud over them because they don't know any other way to be.

Why negativity arises can be because of many reasons. Perhaps experience has taught the individual to expect nothing, though that in itself is a very negative way of looking at life. Perhaps the individual sees their level of luck as being less than zero and won't see the potential of good luck happening in their lives. If I was to tell you that the fortune of an individual is not measured by luck, but by attitude, you would probably think that was a little bit slanted in opinion, but it's actually true. Luck is something that we use as an example when things go either badly or well. It's an adjective but it isn't the reason that things went badly or well. That's largely down to attitude and the level of negativity or positivity.

STEP 1 – BE REALISTIC ABOUT WHO YOU ARE

If you are a negative person, you do need to change your outlook especially if you want to unlock your own potential. Your negativity will hold you back. You need to observe the way that you deal with problems. Chances are that you see the bleak side of things and you need to admit to yourself that you have a problem and that other people around you who are succeeding are doing so not because of luck, but because their attitudes are healthier than yours.

If you are one who blames circumstances for misfortune, then it's time to change that attitude. If you were to walk into an exam room expecting to fail, chances are that you would. Why? Because you don't think yourself capable of passing the exam. With an attitude such as that you are likely to fail. You need to examine the kind of person you are and look at your actions over a period of time to see when you respond to any stimuli in a negative manner. Recognizing the problem is the very first part of being able to do something to change that problem. In this chapter, we are going to give you clues as to how you can change your situation and start to see life in a much more positive way. The steps included in this chapter are straightforward and if you have problems incorporating them into your life at first, make notes and then go on an all-out purge of your old lifestyle, incorporating each and every step that we have given you because it will make a huge difference to the outcome of every situation that you are faced with during the course of your life.

STEP 2 – KEEPING A DAIRY

I ask clients to keep a diary for a purpose. In this diary, they are to keep notes of negative thoughts. Next to each negative thought, they need to write down a potential answer to the problem that gives a positive outcome, thus negating the negativity. For example:

I failed my driving test today

Positive response: I will have more experience next time I take it and I will pass.

My boss gave the best work to my colleague

Positive answer: I will show my boss my capability and next time it will be me that gets given the good work.

My wife does not show her affection

Positive answer: Perhaps if I am more affectionate toward my wife, she will return that affection.

For each negative entry in that book, you need to change your way of thinking to a positive one. This is only background work at this moment in time, but you need a change of attitude if you really do want to succeed and this is the way toward gaining that positivity. People invariably see their failures as being part and parcel of what they can expect in their lives but that depends upon how you look at the disappointments that happen. If you look at them in a negative light and learn nothing from them, then they will only have negative consequences. However, if you write down your negative thoughts and replace them with positive answers, using the failure as your prompt to improve, you can go forward two steps instead of going back and feeling that you are being held back from your dreams.

Each trial in life is a hurdle. It may temporarily stops you from achieving your goals but it isn't have to halt them. Use it so that you go forward with more information and you are more likely to achieve those goals. Use it as a negative giving you fuel for reasons why you fail or justification of a failure, and you learn nothing from it. Look at these case scenarios and you will see what I mean.

- I couldn't win the race because the boy in the next lane was cheating

- I can't have the job that I want because other people always get their first

- I can't possibly reach my goals because there are always going to be those that stand in the way

- I can't have anything good in life because my luck's not that good

These are all excuses used as justification for why you fail. In the first instant the person running was blamed for cheating. In fact, if you were to look at your running skills and do all that you can to improve them, chances are that you could win. Don't use the fortune of others as your justification for failure. In that case, it would have been more appropriate to learn from the other person, rather than accusing him of cheating because it makes you feel instantly better about your own performance. In the case of the job, negative thinking is getting in the way of progression. If you believe that everyone else will come first, you don't even go the extra mile to try for the job. If you really do know that there are other candidates, you need to strengthen your application in a positive manner, rather than accompany it with your own sense of negativity. It may just be that it is your negative attitude that is stopping you from getting the job in the first place. If you really feel that people are getting in the way of your happiness, examine the situation because you are using this as an excuse for your failure. People make choices all the way through their lives. While it's quite possible that you could be held back at some stage of your life by people getting in the way, you need to use this as a lesson and work out a positive conclusion so that next time, they don't. It's all down to you. It's never going to be someone else's fault and if you see it like that, it's usually because you let those people get in your way. You have to find balance and work toward set goals rather than putting off goals assuming that they will be thwarted by others.

As for playing the "luck" card, the next time that you blame "luck" tell yourself that this is absolute nonsense. Yes, occasionally good luck happens but it's not your bad luck that things did not happen to you. There will have been a progression of events that led to this "bad luck" and you need to learn from every rejection in life so that you don't go forward in your life always blaming luck when in fact it is your failure to learn a different approach that is to blame.

STEP 3 – LEARNING ALL ABOUT FOCUS

Did you know that negative thoughts squash all your positive thoughts? Imagine the scenario. You have gone into the forest to admire nature. You had great plans but right now you are standing with a grizzly bear in front of you. What do you do? The chances are that you will focus upon getting away from the bear. You will forget all about the wonderful photo opportunities and certainly won't give much thought to the berries you were thinking of gathering. The reason for this is that negative thoughts take all of your hard work and focus. They detract from anything good. If you let your mind take control of you and keep you in negative mode, you won't experience the joy of success. Of course, if faced by a grizzly bear, you do need to concentrate to this level to get away, but I only used this as an example to show the thought process. The "bear" becomes hypothetical and represents the negative thought that took away the possibility of seeing good things.

Some people go through their lives with a series of "bears" coming into their horizon to spoil the view. If you think in a negative manner each of these negative thoughts represents that bear. If you are angry with someone and stomp off across the park, chances are that you don't see anything in the park. Your mind is too black with anger and the negative thoughts that are going through your mind are blinding you to the possibilities that are out there.

Negative will always beat positive because the thoughts are more urgent and the mind is built in such a way that we concentrate on bad things. If you look at this situation, there are several ways of dealing with it:

Mother in law thinks you are bad at home management

It could be dealt with in two ways. One is the negative way and one concentrates on the positive aspects. The negative person will be concerned about her thoughts and will go out of their way to prove that mother in law is wrong. It becomes the focal point and there isn't room for good thoughts. Thus the mother in law problem becomes huge. She will tidy the whole house, even if the mother in law is only coming for dinner. She will be excessive in her over compensation for bad home management to prove a point to her mother in law. She will concentrate on the negativity that the mother in law is likely to introduce to the event and will not see a positive side to anything surrounding that event. In fact, the way that this individual looks at life is a defensive way. If she feels any criticism from any source, she goes into the offensive and counters it before it actually happens. This is one unhappy lady because she is always centering her life on what other people think of her and the problem is this. While she is so busy trying to compensate for other people's thoughts, she isn't actually enjoying life very much.

The other way is to focus on the positive. Mother in law doesn't live in the same house and that means you don't have to live with the criticism. Don't sweat it. It's only going to be a short visit and then she can go home to her home where she is in control of home management.

It sounds easier said than done, but if you put your focus always on the positive, you get through difficult situations unscathed. You don't have to concentrate all your energies on bad things and you can move forward, show mother in law your positivity and perhaps it will rub off on her. If it doesn't, it's her problem – not yours. You cannot control the opinions of others, but you can control the way that you let their opinions rule your life and dictate your level of happiness.

Focus on the positive side of every situation because if you want to succeed in life, you have to start seeing the cup as half full, and not let the opinions of others hamper your ambitions. Look in your workplace at the girl who gets accused of not pulling her weight. If she is the cup half empty type of person, work will be a very miserable place for her because she feels she is not living up to expectations. However, if she is the cup half full type of person, she won't really be that bothered about what other people think and can remain positive, knowing that what she does is what she is capable of.

The focus that you put onto the negative changes everything. If you are always looking for fault, you will always find it because your mind is making it happen. If, for example, I were to check on the housework to make sure that it is done correctly, I will find dust. However, if I take the house at face value and enjoy it regardless of that little speck of dust I am the winner. It's not that the house is dirty. It's the negative person who seeks to find dirt where other people don't even notice. Stop being the one to create problems in your own life and in the lives of people around you. Be positive and see things from a positive viewpoint. Let's show you a ridiculous case of concentration on the negative so that you can see how foolish you are being to yourself and the people that matter to you. Focus on good things helps you to enjoy your lot in life and in the next demonstrations, we will take a situation and dissect it into two sections. One man sees everything in a positive light. The other is totally negative and perhaps the example is a little extreme, but it is like that for a purpose – to show you how focusing on the negative spoils everything.

Scenario 1 – Negative focus. A man goes into a restaurant and orders an 8oz steak. When it arrives, it looks a little on the skinny side and he complains very loudly that the steak looks less than 8 ounces. The waiter doesn't know what to do but the man is so adamant that the steak is undersized that he is making a spectacle of himself in front of paying customers. He is invited to the kitchen. He is shown a pile of steaks and the chef puts one onto the scales to show him that all the steaks are indeed 8oz steaks. However, he is not satisfied. He takes his own steak from the plate, scrapes the gravy off and places it onto the scales and it's less than 8 oz. The chef explains that as a steak cooks, it loses some of its weight. The man feels that he has been cheated and insists that the chef cooks him a fresh 8oz steak from the pile which is weighed in advance. He watches it being cooked. He sits back in his place and is served with the steak and eats it, even though he has a feeling in the back of his mind that the original steak was a short measure and he even has the thought in his mind that this steak may not be the one that the chef showed him going into the pan. Negative thoughts are ridiculous. They take away the enjoyment of life. This man was so busy thinking of the weight of the steak and the fact that he thought he was being cheated that he didn't even taste it very much. His thoughts were too occupied with focusing on the negative.

Scenario 2 – Positive focus – We will use the same scenario but we will change the character in the scenario. In this case, a man is served with his steak. He smells the aroma and enjoys the taste and texture of the steak. It's wonderfully easy to cut and tastes absolutely delicious. He enjoys the taste of the vegetables that the chef has chosen and thinks that the meal is a very positive experience. People who are sitting with the man are happy to be in his company because of his positive attitude. He feels happy with the meal and the company that he is in.

The difference between the two situations is clear. Those who were dining with the angry man would have been embarrassed by his behavior while those who mixed with the positive man would be very impressed by being in his company.

Although the above scene is a little extreme, you need to see it in black and white that what you focus on in life is what you are going to get. If you see the world as being a place where everything is negative – it becomes negative. If you focus on the positive, however, everything changes. You become a magnate for friendships, you are able to reap the benefits of the law of attraction and good things happen to you. That focus is imperative. Even when faced with difficult situations, you let your positive side see something that can be gained from the worst scenario you can imagine because you will have trained your mind to always err on the side of positivity.

If you can consciously look at the bad things that happen during the course of the days that follow and try to see the positive slant, you begin to see things in a very different way and it is this that you have to foster if you really want abundance in your life. There is no meat for dinner – never mind – we can experiment with new vegetables and taste something new. The car won't start. Never mind, it will do us good to walk. Focus on the good side of everything because when you learn to do that, you are able to go through life as a much happier person. Your focus in life determines the outcome and that's what you will begin to see as you begin to focus on the positive.

Look at people around you who seem to be successful and happy. Do they focus on the negative? If they do, then the situation that they are in at that given time will be a negative situation that will take away the shine of their success. Use role models who are positive and whose attitude shines because once you can start doing that, good things will start to happen in your life.

STEP 4 – BEING POSITIVE IN EVERYTHING

People who allow the negative side of life to create barriers will always blame fate for things not happening as they wished. In fact, if you pass blame to circumstance or to other people, you are doing things the wrong way. Learn from life to see things in a positive way. If a car you wanted to buy is sold to someone else, it isn't a bad thing. It just means that you were not meant to buy that car. New doors will open to you when you are able to view life in this way. See opportunity – it is there if you look hard enough.

I remember being terribly upset that I was not able to buy a home that I had set my heart on. I continually thought about it and it clouded my judgment for quite a while. In fact, I saw the negative side of everything because of that one incident. What I was unaware of was that when I got over it and started to look again for a suitable house, without that constant nagging in the back of my mind, I actually found one that was better and doors started to open instead of keeping firmly closed in front of me. You blinker your own opportunities by dwelling on the negative. When you step away from the negative, you see things in a clearer way and are able to glean other opportunities that are even better than your original one.

There was a very old movie where Walt Disney presented the story of a young girl, Pollyanna, who saw the positive side of every situation. Although the movie was a made for children, it actually had a very valid message in that it showed viewers how everything changes when you can see the possibility, rather than the disadvantages that life offers you. You need to see the bright side of every situation and learn to be grateful for things that come out of that bad situation. When you are able to do this, you have less setbacks in life and don't get so negative about things. If you want to know the benefit of positive thinking, you need to use it in every situation that life throws at you.

There is a positive side to every event that happens in your life and although some will bring out sadness, there is always going to be a positive spin that you can put on any situation at all. As I am writing this, sadness has enfolded me through the loss of a very close friend, but I am able to use my positivity to think myself very fortunate indeed to have had that friend who has set me many examples in my life and who has enriched my life. Even the direst of circumstances can bring out positivity if you let it. Make a conscious effort to examine the things that happen in your life and put some kind of positive spin on them because that teaches you what strength you can gain in moments of sadness and potential weakness. This helps you to cope with life and to be happier but it also teaches you the benefits of humility and empathy.

CHAPTER TWO

KNOW WHAT YOU WANT OUT OF LIFE

I once knew someone who said that they wanted to be rich. I asked "How rich?" and they thought that this question was a weird question. It wasn't. If you have vague ambitions, you get varied and often vague results. You have to envision what you actually want in life in order to work toward it. It's like getting into a car and not knowing where you are going if you don't envision what would make you successful and what would make you happy. There are people who are very successful at using the law of attraction to get the things that they need, want or desire. If you go onto websites such as YouTube and type in Law of attraction, you will see that there are thousands of stories about people who use this to get what they want out of life. There are even lottery winners who believed to such an extent that they would win the lottery that they actually did. One woman even visualized her win and knew exactly how much it was that she was going to win and that was the exact amount of her lottery check. What you are doing when you know what you are aiming at is make the target of your life clearer, so that you work toward it. You are giving your life a destination. Think of life as a car journey and you are more likely to reach the destination if it is planned out and you know where you are going.

For just one moment, close your eyes and think of all the things that make you sad. The reason I am asking you to do this is because visualization is very powerful indeed. If you want to make yourself cry, the visualization of sad things that really did tug on your heartstrings can bring those tears on and make you cry. You can even visualize sad events in your life by listening to music that brings you back to that sad time. Why would you want to do that? Some people do it to relive bad times because they can't quite get beyond them. In this particular case, I am asking you to do it just to demonstrate how powerful the mind is and how powerful your own visualizations are. If you want to be unhappy, then sad thoughts will do it for you. However, if you want to be happy and successful, they won't. Thus you need to tune into thoughts that are positive and that reinforce the dreams that you want to become a reality.

STEP 5 – KNOW YOUR DREAMS

Write down what you want to achieve. When you see it on paper, you reinforce the ambition. Now read what you wrote and close your eyes. Imagine that you have that thing that you want to be in your life. See yourself with it. See the difference that it makes to your life. This is called visualization. You may not believe in it, but you need to start changing your view. The fact is that it has been proven to work. If you look on YouTube at people who won the lottery, they did so because they had a belief that they could win and in some cases even predicted the exact amount that they would win, as previously stated. One woman went to bed with the amount written on a piece of paper under her pillow and that was the exact amount that she won. This uses the Power of

Attraction and that's a very powerful magnet to get what it is that you want. So how do you start this kind of visualization? You need to have a dream. You need to be able to see yourself in a set situation and be able to feel that situation as being real. For example, if you want to buy a villa in Italy, visualize it. See it and feel the sunshine against your skin. Add all the detail to the image. There could be vineyards or there could be canals and lakes. Your vision is yours and no one else's. Don't dream for other people. Those that do this often get it wrong because they see their partner's dream as being totally different from how their partner sees it. If you have friends where one of spouse has bought tickets for a vacation that the other was disappointed in, that's because his image is different to hers or vice versa.

If you want to be a successful writer, see yourself at work. See the pages unfold. See the acceptance letter from a publishing company. Envisage the success of the book. Your dream is your own and no one can ever take that away from you and the more detail you can add to that vision, the more likely it is that it will work. The thing is that you are using the same part of the brain in which memories are stored. If you were to think back to a happy event in your life, you would be able to visualize it just as it happened. When you are working on positive attitude and visualizations, you are creating the picture that you want to form part of your future. That gives you something to aim at in your life that may otherwise not have been there. People with aims and goals in life tend to reach them easier than those people who don't visualize success or happiness. Therefore, you need to work on that image.

Over the course of time your visualizations will change and be adapted because of new facets added to that dream. People change and so must the dream goal because age will change what you want out of life and new visualizations help you to keep all those dreams and hopes current, so that they are actually relevant to your life in this day and age. Here, maybe I should explain why people adjust their visualizations. If you were to visualize yourself on a beach in the sunshine, who's to say that your tastes will not change and evolve over time? People who enjoy the beach at one phase of their lives may see other things as more enjoyable as they grow older. Thus keeping your visualizations up to date is the way that you help yourself to move toward the most current goals.

STEP 6 – WORKING TOWARD YOUR DREAMS

When you know what you are aiming for, it's a lot easier to achieve it. Thus, you need to try and plan your way forward and take each step of the way as it comes to you. Instead of seeing things are becoming hurdles, see them as being there for a reason. Perhaps you need to refine your wish list and make it go in a different direction to make your dreams come true. Never see diversions as anything other than that which they are. Never see the negative side of rejection or changes in direction, because if you believe that there is always a reason why things change, you can still keep your eye on your eventual goals and reach them. Perhaps you have a bucket list of things that you would like to achieve. If you were to share this with your spouse, chances are that your spouse also has dreams that he/she wants to achieve. You open up the possibility of those things happening if you are able to discuss them as well as visualizing them. Although one of the tips in this book is about sharing your dreams, in this case we are talking about personal ambitions. Perhaps you want to go and see the Northern Lights but you know that your partner is not interested. By showing an interest in his bucket list and learning more about what he likes, you are opening the door to having your dreams recognized by your partner. It's much more likely that your dream will come true if you have already introduced the subject and your partner knows that this is a personal ambition that you have always wanted to achieve.

Working toward your dreams can mean saving. Perhaps your dreams cost money that you don't have but when you decide to work toward them, you have more incentive to stop spending on frivolous things that don't enhance your life at all and put that money into other priorities which help you to fulfill your wish list of things to do. The point is that if you have dreams and do not work your way toward them, then they are not going to happen.

A lady friend of mine wanted to become a published poet. She had always written poetry and could certainly write them well, though she had never shared the dream with anyone or done anything toward making that dream come true. When she brought up the subject to her husband one night, he made the suggestion that she put time aside to collect up her poems and get them into shape to send to a publisher. Inadvertently, by mentioning her dream to her husband, she had started that dream in motion. He could see how much it meant to her and was prepared to adjust their lives to make sure that she had the time to fit in the time she needed to prepare her manuscript. When she did get rejected, she didn't give up or feel negative about it. In fact, her husband had warned her to be prepared for rejection. She just needed to find the right publishing house that was looking for the kind of work that she was producing and eventually found it. You don't get there by letting rejection make you think negatively. You don't get there by letting obstacles get in the way of your belief in your dream. However, you do get there if you continue to calmly visualize your work in print or whatever your dream is and continue to work toward it.

There are other things that you can do if your dreams involve different aspects of your life that could be worked on. Those wanting to buy a home abroad, for example, could complement their dream by learning the language of the people that live in that country. It's making things more concrete and it's making yourself more qualified to enjoy the dream when it happens. Someone who wants to be a racing driver needs to have more contact with people in that field so that opportunities open up that wouldn't open up if it was simply a wish. You need to believe in your dream, to visualize it on a regular basis, but you also need to put in the effort to help make that dream come true.

STEP 7 – MOTIVATING YOURSELF

When you have dreams in mind and are working toward them, you need to keep your motivation consistent. If you lose that motivation, you step two steps backward instead of forward. Even if things do not go in the way that you planned, think that there must be a positive reason for that change in the plan and motivate yourself using what you learned. Motivation has a lot to do with success. If someone wants to succeed at something badly enough and have sufficient motivation, they are likely to work toward that goal, regardless of obstacles that get in the way.

You need to look at the cases of athletes who are disabled. They didn't feel sorry for themselves. They didn't stop their lives mid track, though they could have done and no one would have blamed them for it. Instead, they found the motivation inside themselves to carry on against all odds and succeed. Your motivation level should always be positive because that's what drives you and gives you the impetus to succeed.

In the last couple of tips, we told you about working toward your dreams and visualizing the dream coming true. Sometimes this is sufficient to keep the motivation going. At low points, and we all have them, try to have inspiration around you that will lift you out of the pits in life and make you doubt your dreams. Your dreams are as valid as anyone else's but you will have to work toward them. Think of negativity as taking you away from them.

Think of the tide on the shore pulling you away from that final goal with a power that you have no control over and that's what your negativity will do to you. Avoid negativity at all costs.

STEP 8 – BELIEVE IN YOURSELF

When you are chasing your dreams, you have to believe in yourself completely. If you look at historical cases, you can see how this works. Bill Gates believed in the possibility of Windows and went to a bank to ask for financial help in the early stages of his beliefs. Imagine how he would have felt had he taken the rejection seriously and given up on his dreams. He believed in himself and in his dream and look where that got his company. You need to believe in yourself regardless of what others think because it is this belief that will give you the boost of energy you need to walk forward into success. If your dream is real enough to you, it's real enough to hold onto and part of that realization comes from believing in yourself. Life sends all kinds of trials. These may make you feel bad about life but they should never make you feel bad about who you are. Belief in yourself comes from being true to how you feel instead of putting up pretention just because you feel you need to. You don't. The authentic self that is the core part of your belief system is what keeps you strong and makes you a happier person. I once asked someone how they had continued toward their dream when so many bad things had happened in that person's life. I had never seen such negative events all happen to one person and it was her belief in herself that kept her believing in that dream eventually one day coming true. She was always true to herself – even when this went against popular opinion and that was her core strength and what took her toward achievement of her dreams. It was a long road, but with her belief in herself intact, she knew that it was only a matter of time before things changed. Belief in yourself helps you to get past all the obstacles that are placed in your path.

It is also all that you need to help you to keep your goals on track. If you believe that you will achieve something, even if it is an eventual goal, you have somewhere to aim and you are much more likely to achieve your goal.

STEP 9 – RE-ASSESSING YOUR DREAMS

If your dream changes, it's evolving. It doesn't mean that one dream died a death. It means that you adjusted the dream as you learned something new that may have made the dream more viable. Don't be afraid of change. As you grow older, your ambitions change and perhaps the dream evolves into something entirely different because of life changes that happened. Go with it and trust your instincts because they are rarely wrong.

The reason I say this is because in one case that I can cite, a young man had goals to run in marathons. He loved running and the sense of freedom that it gave him was amazing. Crippled in an accident, he stayed true to himself and still saw running as a real possibility although of course, he had to adjust the dream in order for him to keep it on track. That same person began to run marathons for the disabled and found that same level of enjoyment and satisfaction from what he was doing, even though an adjustment had to be made.

Others have adjusted their dreams to take account of changing circumstances instead of simply giving up and blaming life for the dream not being able to come true. If you want to live in a house that's wonderful and then find yourself unable to walk up the stairs as you get older, adjust the dream because there are just as wonderful places that don't have stairs. If you dream involves something that life won't allow you to do, adjust it so that you can achieve it. People who give up because of circumstance tend to blame life for getting in the way, though it wasn't life that got in the way. It was the limited scope of their dreams. Dreams expand and contract. They can be tailored to your needs but there is no reason on earth why they have to be abandoned simply because of a change in circumstance.

When you think of great composers who even continued to compose wonderful music when they were deaf or painters who lost their hands and had to adapt to using their feet, it's obvious that adjustment needs to be made to dreams to fit the reality that you are living in and this adjustment may be all that you need to make the dream come true. Your thought processes change with every second that passes but if your dreams are consistent and strongly felt, you can always find a way to fulfill them by being flexible in your approach. Let your dream grow with you. Keep true to yourself and let the dream evolve because often that dream can be fulfilled faster when you are able to adjust it to your circumstances.

One of the most common reasons why people do not fulfil their dreams or find true happiness is because they allow obstacles to put an end to dreams. They use blame of people or blame of circumstances as the reasons that the dream could not be fulfilled and when you do this, you introduce a new facet into your life that is not related to success or happiness. That facet is bitterness. It is regret and resentment. I once spoke to a client whose bitterness and resentment were so strong that they overpowered any thought of getting his dream back on track. I asked him how he felt about this and his answers showed me how he had not understood that dreams can be altered to fit circumstances:

- It was his fault because he ruined my chances of ever being happy

- It was getting on the wrong side of fate

- I hate life for what it has done to me

You may read the stories of victims in the newspapers or online and feel very sorry for people whose sadness comes from shattered dreams, but what these people are not appreciating is that the only reason that dreams die is because you allow them to. Circumstance cannot kill dreams unless you let it. Another person cannot kill your dreams unless you allow them to. You are an island and always will be and on this island, you have many opportunities to go in a positive direction of a negative one. When things happen, they may make the dream a little more distant, but if you have belief in self and a belief in the dream – you will be able to adjust it and still allow it to come true.

CHAPTER THREE

UNDERSTANDING HOW THE BRAIN WORKS

The brain works in a very logical way and I believe that if you know how it is likely to react to any given circumstance, you can give your mind the advantage and get to where you want to go in a quicker way. In this chapter we discover the kind of things that can hold you back and give readers ideas about how to tackle these and to make them happen less often in their lives. If you understand the way that the brain works, this enables you to be able to step in and make the brain work in a different way, knowing that the chain of thoughts that goes through the mind is quite logical. The mindset with which you control your life will dictate whether your life or events in it have a positive or negative outcome.

You have much more control over your life than you think you have. If you suffer from depression or are easily made to feel inferior, you need to be able to work on your character and this is only a matter of practicing positive exercises that allow you to see things in a different light, so that you can remain positive, even when negative things happen. You are in the driving seat of your life until such time as you relinquish that position. Giving up or being negative is an option, but it's only an option. It's a choice that only you can make but when you choose to go the negative way, you negate your own dreams and sabotage your own chances at finding happiness.

STEP 10 – UNDERSTANDING THE EFFECT OF NEGATIVE THOUGHTS

In experiments, scientists put groups of people into different settings. Some were given positive things to look at, some negative and some neutral. They were then asked to give feedback. The brain picks up on positive thoughts. In the group that were fed positivity, plenty of ideas came forward. In the neutral group, people had a few ideas but nothing special and in the negative group, there was very little that the participants could put on their pieces of paper because the negativity had wiped out any creativity they may otherwise have had. This proves conclusively that negative thoughts stand in the way of your dreams.

Try it for yourself if you don't believe in the impact of negativity. Present yourself with the mediocre and your creativity level drops. Present yourself with the dynamic, and you start to work toward your dreams. Present yourself with the neutral and you go neither forward nor backward and are unlikely to reach your dreams in this manner because it takes real effort on your part to make them come true.

Thus, you can see from this that brain works on the stimulus that it is given. If you want to be happy and have everything going your way, you need to surround yourself with sufficient stimulation to keep the dreams alive. When you place children into a barren environment but give them sufficient materials to create something, they will amaze you. The furtive minds of children have not yet let negativity spoil their creative ideas and from a cardboard box, they can produce a magical castle or from pieces of wood, they can produce the sword that will slay the dragon. Keep yourself creative at all times by allowing your brain all of the food that it needs to do this. If you are artistically inclined, have the materials available so you can explore your art. If you think that you would be good at doodling, you won't be much good if you can't find a crayon and paper. You need to keep yourself motivated. You may wonder where artistic talents come in the order of things, but the creative side of the brain allows people to come up with ideas and that's where dreams are brewed. Keep your creative side active because it fires the imagination and helps you to envision your dream and to keep it in the motivational area of your mind.

STEP 11 – FEEDING THE BRAIN POSITIVITY

If you want success in your life, then you need to feed yourself with positive attitude. Positivity drives success. It drives new ideas. In fact, in large multi-million dollar businesses, entrepreneurs are encouraged to strive for a happy work environment where people's needs are met because this makes the workers more productive and energetic. This means that what they produce will be more than what would be produced in a negative environment. Feed your brain positivity. Tell yourself that you can succeed and believe it.

The way to reinforce positivity is to set yourself goals that are small at first and that you know that you can manage, making them gradually more difficult as time passes. You need goals that make you strive, rather than silly goals that give you no real sense of achievement although if you have self-esteem problems or do not have faith in yourself, start them as manageable goals and work on toward more difficult ones. What you are doing is feeding your brain positive affirmation that you are capable of working toward these goals and when you achieve one of them, celebrate it in some small way.

Goals can be anything. They can be writing a list of small tasks you know you have been putting off and doing them all, ticking each one of them with a sense of satisfaction once it has been achieved. It can be weight loss goals, goals for doing household tasks, goals to get in touch by telephone with old friends that you have been neglecting or anything at all. List things out and work out how hard a goal you can manage at this point in time and then gradually make them harder so you have to really work to get there. The difference between attaining an easy goal and one that you have to work at is that the harder one will give you a much fuller sense of achievement once it is reached.

STEP 12 – GETTING RID OF NEGATIVE TOXINS

Have you ever heard of toxins? These are things that are detrimental to a positive environment. Toxicity can also apply to relationships. If you have people within your life that hold you back by feeding you too much negativity, you need to work out if these people have a place in your life. Friends who are toxic are those who are always negative and always feeding you negativity. If you want to be successful and happy, surround yourself with successful and happy people. That doesn't mean dropping the poor relatives. Poor people can be very positive. It means choosing your friends wisely and deciding which friends believe in your sufficiently to offer you positive support.

To help you to decide which friends are the ones you want to keep and the ones you should consider dropping, ask yourself which friends are constantly using you but give very little back to the relationship. These are toxic friends and they obviously have little respect for you. They may ask you to babysit on a regular basis or expect you to do their running around for them all of the time. That's fine if they are people who are unable to do these things, but often users are very capable of doing their own dirty work but just prefer to get someone else to do it.

Other negative toxins may be in the foods that you eat. Eat fresh food and let your body get the maximum from the diet that you eat. Make it varied and interesting. It takes a little longer to cook food from fresh but try a few stir fries Chinese style as these are really quick to prepare and don't have all the chemicals in them that bought and prepared foods do.

If you are a smoker, try to stop smoking and replace it with patches if you need the nicotine. Open the windows and air your home to ensure that you home is toxin free. If you live in an environment that is damp, try to do something about it because all of the toxins that you take into your body could be because of the environment you live in. Sometimes fixing things like this makes the world of difference. These may be toxins in your environment, toxic friendships or even toxic behavior on your part but you need to detox your life to get the best benefit from it and to enable yourself to think positively.

STEP 13 – FEEDING YOUR BRAIN POSITIVITY

Some of the best coaches on the Internet will tell you that you need to work on your dream 7 days a week. Even if only a small portion of weekend days is used in working toward your dream, keeping up the positive attitude and the hard work will pay off. You cannot believe in yourself for five days a week and then drop it for two. You need your brain to stay in positive mode at all times. If you find something is stopping you from feeling positive, you need to make changes. When you are working toward a set dream that means putting everything that you have into that work. You may find yourself thinking out new ideas on your days off. That's fine too because it's firing up the imagination ready for the new working week. You need to see positivity in action to actually keep up your belief in it. Look how others gain their positivity. There are loads of entrepreneurs and coaches online and the clues are there. One of the biggest clues is believing in yourself no matter how far out there your dream appears to be to others. Belief in yourself is huge when it comes to achieving your goals in life. You don't get stopped in your route by self-doubt and you don't allow what others say to initiate self-doubt because you are so sure of your own ability to fulfill your goals.

Does that mean you won't have unproductive days? Of course it doesn't. Everyone needs a certain amount of rest, but make that rest quality time for your brain. You may have things that you want to do or may even want to be pampered on your days off. Go for it and enjoy it. You deserve it.

STEP 14 – FEEDING YOUR BRAIN

As we know that creativity is driven by positivity, you need to feed your brain a good supply of positive creative tasks. These could be making plans toward meeting new people. They could be getting into creative mode by traditional art fields. Whatever you feed your mind in a creative way helps to drive positivity and will help you to reach your dreams. All of the time that you are feeding your brain with creativity, you are reinforcing that positivity is part of who you are. That doesn't mean you will be good at everything that you try, but by adjusting your thinking, you can feed your brain by saying the following:

Well – I learned today that painting isn't my forte. That gives me other ideas to pursue.

Rather than

I was a failure and I made a real mess of painting.

You have to stop seeing failure. The fact that you cannot do everything isn't failure. It is merely a question of eliminating things that really don't float your boat. It's not a negative thing that everyone in the world isn't good at calligraphy. If they were, calligraphy would have very little value. Find your niche and enjoy it and feed your mind as much positivity as you can, even if you perceive failure. It isn't failure. It's simply discovering something new about yourself.

The other things that help you to stay focused are brain teasers such as crossword puzzles, or even the odd computer game that reinforces your brain power. Luminosity is one of these and it allows you to exercise your brain on a daily basis. It's fun and even if you don't get all the answers correct, it gives you something to aim at. Your mind does need a certain amount of recreation. Whatever you choose, make sure that it's something that you enjoy doing and that helps you to stretch your mind. While some may find joy in a jigsaw puzzle, your joy may be solving something more complex but only you can say what kind of activity will stretch your mind. Keeping active and keeping the brain working is all part and parcel of keeping yourself fit.

Feed your brain with positive input. Whenever you manage to do something, make sure that your brain feels congratulated for it. If you fail to do something, don't feed your brain failure. Get your brain to work on another way of achieving whatever it was that you failed at. You won't always get things right first time but when you do, the sense of victory is much stronger if you initially failed in your effort. Imagine a task that is hard to do. Then use the brain to solve the problem. When it eventually does solve it, it's positivity that the mind feels. You feel smug and you have every right to. What many people make the mistake of doing is feeding their minds negativity because of failure, when in fact failure is just one step toward success.

- I need to change the locks on the window
- This method does not work, so I need to find another method that does

This is the attitude to feed your mind because you are still working in a positive manner even though the first method did not work. In fact, you are heading toward the goal with more information – not less – and this should help you to solve the equation. It's a much better attitude than saying:

- I need to change the locks on the window

- This method doesn't work. Why am I so stupid?

And yet, so many people see their failures as the end of the story. It's only the end of the story if you allow it to be and even if you have to employ professionals to fix the window lock at the end of the day, the problem has been dealt with successfully. Don't assume you have to do everything. You are not superwoman or superman but with a change of attitude and by feeding your brain good information, you could be!

CHAPTER FOUR

FINDING THE THINGS YOU LOVE TO DO

If you want to be happy and successful, then finding the things you love to do and doing them will do the trick. However, it's not as easy as that in the initial stages. You need to work toward those aims. Let's see how you can start to glean success and happiness at the same time by doing what you love. There are various steps that lead you toward this and you can't skimp on these. Whether you want to do things simply for the pleasure of doing them or to eventually make a living, you still need the right approach. Think of people like writer, J. J. Rawlins or even J. R. Tolkien. These are people who made an absolute fortune from their own imaginations – doing things that they enjoyed. Although Tolkien didn't live to see his books being turned into movies, he had the right idea and developed it and was able to make his living using something that was in his imagination. Not everyone can do that but you can work toward doing the things that you love to do and learning to incorporate them into your life.

STEP 15 – DECIDE WHAT YOU DO LOVE

This isn't just something that you like. It's something that you have a passion about. Write down the things that you would love to do for a living. For instance, if you like kids, then perhaps working with kids would give you the greatest amount of pleasure. If you like writing, then perhaps this would be the right avenue for you. Your success depends not just on how much you earn, but how happy and passionate you feel about the way that you earn. You need to create a shortlist of things that you really derive pleasure from. These will give you clues as to the direction you need to be going in. For example, typical things that people feel passionate about could be painting, interior design, hairdressing, makeup, exercise of some kind, country walking, pony riding, etc. The scope is very wide because all different people will have different ideas as to what their passion is. This isn't just something that you like. It's something that you have a passion for. A walker, for example, may have a passion for being out in the countryside and breathing in fresh air as well as seeing the changes of the season.

Someone who loves hairdressing may like to put their skills to work because it's a passion and she/he knows that it improves people's lives. If you love exercise, and I mean love it as opposed to liking it, perhaps you feel the adrenalin and that gives you the buzz that makes you happy. Since there are so many choices to make, think small at first. Close your eyes and think about the things you do that bring you that amount of pleasure and then list them and see if there is a way that you can incorporate these into your life path as a potential career. An ex pat living in a foreign country was so tired of only having the potential to do lousy jobs. Her immigrant status only allowed her to work in factories or stores and she wanted more for herself. Her passion was baking and she made the most heavenly cupcakes. By finding out about the market, she was able to set herself up as the cupcake lady and sell these wonderful cakes in fancy boxes and make her living at it. The nice thing for her was that she was able to experiment with new tastes and flavors and introduce new lines each week to see which turned out to be favorites with her customers. This was an idea borne of necessity, but it meant that she spent her life doing something that she truly loved and positive thinking helps you to do this. When you identify that which gives you joy, you can then look further and see how this joy can be turned into a regular thing to enhance the life that you have.

STEP 16 – LOOKING FOR VIABLE WORK WITHIN YOUR AREA OF PASSION

The trouble with people today is that they settle for less than they actually want to do. They feel that they cannot succeed in the areas where their passions lie. However, people do make a living doing what they love every day of the week. A writer, for example, can begin writing for companies that pay for that writing. It may not be the type of writing that the person wants to do as their eventual aim, but it leads them into the right direction. Someone who loves scuba diving may not have the finance to open a scuba diving club but they may still be able to work in one until opportunity presents itself. In both of these cases, the individual will be doing what he/she wants to do and learning to be better at it all of the time, so that when the eventual dream happens, they are ready for it.

Of course, you may not equate making the dream come true with having to work, but unfortunately, realistically, you have to live while you search for that perfect niche. If that means working for someone else and proving yourself, then that's okay because you will still be doing the work that makes you feel passionate and creative. If you have a passion for cars, it won't matter to you whether you are working for a garage for your monthly salary or whether you are working on a project for yourself because the passion itself is cars. Thus try to make a path for yourself toward your eventual aim and make sure that the work that takes you there is something that really does fire up your passion.

Often people who are passionate about something interview just as well as those who are overly qualified. Believe with all of your heart that this is the road that you want to take and show the world what you are made of. Reporters don't all go through university. Just once in a while a newspaper gives a reporter a chance to work based upon their enthusiasm and ability to write. You need to believe in your own passions sufficiently to have a good sense of being able to persuade others. When you do, this opens doors for you. Don't expect every door to open. Look for plenty of doors so that you always have an alternative. People who put all of their hope into one thing are those that come unstuck when that one thing fails. Instead of doing that, think of loads of possibilities that could lead you to where you want to be. The lady who wanted to run her own gym didn't have any ideas about giving gym classes to seniors, but that was the only opening there was and she saw it as a gateway to doing something more in line with her dream and took the opportunity.

As it happened, it was only a year before an opening within the same franchise became available which was exactly what she was looking for. You have to keep your belief in yourself alive and keep on looking for the opportunities that are out there – because they are. They become unavailable when you stop believing in them.

STEP 17 – LEARNING MORE ABOUT YOUR PASSION

The more you can learn about those things that you feel passionate about, the more likely you are to be able to make your future built around those passions. We never know everything, but we can feed ourselves so much positivity so that instead of seeing our future as a dream, we can actually watch it start to happen. That's what's so great about having so much enthusiasm for your dream. This enthusiasm gives you motivation and in turn motivation keeps you hungry for more. For example, if you know that you need qualifications to head you in a certain direction, find out what they are and see if you are able to take part time courses that will help you to get there. If you can't go for courses, what online qualifications are there that may be considered? You need to learn more about what you would be expected to do if you were in your dream job and having more knowledge is always going to help you to get your foot in the door.

One man wanted to work as a personal trainer. He thought that he had something very valuable to offer. When he worked out what he was offering to people, he added different elements so that his coaching work would help him to appeal to a wider cross section of people. All of this enthusiasm came from a background of being bullied when he was a kid and his initial aim was to help kids in this situation. However, his dream evolved and he was able to see there were other behavioral problems experienced by young adults that he could learn about. By the time his business was set up, he was able to make sufficient money from his coaching to actually free up time to give free coaching to the kids who were experiencing bullying. The point is that somewhere along the line, you can get back to the root purpose of your direction and he used his abilities to do just that.

The more you learn about your passion, the more you are able to pass on to others. Learning guitar was one of my passions and the more I learned, the more I was able to pass on to people who have never picked up a guitar before. I learned chords, barre chords, picking etc. and the more I was able to learn, the more people I was able to teach in different styles of guitar work, making the potential of teaching much more viable. It's not enough to have a set passion. You need to expand upon that passion and make it into something that will positively benefit others. When you do, it will start to positively benefit you as well.

You may find in the course of your investigation into your passion that it leads to other passions and that's okay too. Keep your research positive. Go in a direction that you feel is right for you. One man was interested in working with a specific variety of dog which he thought was his passion. As he investigated openings even more thoroughly, he actually found that his passion changed midstream as he was introduced to another breed that he found more fascinating. If you look into your area of passion and find yourself pulled into another direction, don't be concerned about it. Go with the flow because there may be doors waiting to open that you don't yet know about.

The doors to opportunity wait for those who are willing to look for them. If you fail at one thing, stay positive and know that there must a cosmic reason why that didn't happen, rather than it being your own personal failure. Don't use disappointment to fire negative thoughts about your passions because that's when your ambitions end and the doors firmly close in your face. You have to believe in what you are doing and even when one door closes, be ready for the next one which may open in the near future. Life isn't about taking one steady straight line. Sometimes you find yourself going off at tangents, but then find that there were good reasons why that happened.

STEP 18 – LEARNING TO BALANCE CONFLICTS

This is one of the biggest hurdles that you will face in life. There may be difficult times where your work and home life balance is out of whack. You need to have distinct areas for both and make sure that your partner is every bit as enthusiastic about your dream as you are. That way, this will diminish the conflict to a certain extent because your partner will have more understanding about why you work such long hours. You do need leisure time though, so you have to learn how to make compromises that work both in favor of your home life and your working life.

If you are working toward doing what you love, you need to find a balance whereby your work can fit with your home life. Many professions these days can be done from home and perhaps it's time to investigate what you can do to help restore that balance as it will help you to become more successful but also happier. Remember too that your partner may not be accustomed to having you around 24 hours a day and may want his/her personal space respected. That's okay too because that helps to fuel a personal relationship with enthusiasm. I can cite mistakes that people make when they change the course of their lives and you may see from this that there are mistakes that you can avoid.

Amy and her partner William decided that they wanted to go and live overseas. Both had their careers to think about and although they argued about how it would work for a long time, they decided that they could do it and both could follow their passions. The reality was a lot different. They found that they were isolated to a certain extent as they did not speak the language and they were not accustomed to spending 24 hours a day together, even though doing their separate work via the Internet. It caused a lot of problems within their relationship and it was decided that the way forward was to look at all the conflicts of interest and work their way through them, so that at the end of the day, their dream was still intact. The kind of things that they found difficult were:

- Being away from family

- Not having friends

- Having no private time away from their partner

- They had problems with the local language

- Living what seemed to be a domesticated life instead of the exotic life they had pictured

They resolved all of this by being truthful about it. Amy was able to gain a little independence from William by taking regular trips home and arranging trips for relatives so that they didn't lose touch with people who were important to them. They made a concerted effort to get out and about and to join social clubs that suited their interests. Her interests were different to his, so that meant that they each followed their own passions and made friends within those passions, thus widening their social circle and learning the language at the same time. As their learning of the language became more proficient, their life in that country opened up because you only see half of the picture if you don't speak the language of the natives. The exotic life that they had envisioned became a reality but it took a lot of work on their part to make this happen.

Conflicts will happen and you don't have to give up a relationship that is otherwise healthy just to pursue your dream. You have to work on conflict resolution and make your dream fit into your lifestyle so that it suits everyone. There are thousands of people worldwide that are doing just this and it is successful because consideration is given to all the family and each are permitted to chase their own dreams within the safety net of the family, rather than being pushed aside so that one person can live their dream.

STEP 19 – USING POSITIVITY TO HELP YOU TO KEEP YOUR OPTIONS OPEN

Never narrow your own possibilities by being so fixed on your dream that you don't see the bigger picture. If you have the chance to learn something new, this can fill the void in your life and help you to shape your dreams. You may be unhappy now because you really don't know what your dream is. By continuing to strive and learn and putting positive energy into it, you can find that dream and can achieve it.

You may not know it yet, but the ideal solution for your life may be waiting around the corner. If you never look that far, how will you find it? You need to start with an idea of something that drives you and something you feel passionate about. Then you need to look into ways that you can incorporate that dream into your life so that it becomes an everyday event. If it takes time to actually work toward that dream, it doesn't matter. Positive thinking helps you to begin to plant roots for that idea. You will find that your ideas change but that's okay as well but you are using your positive attitude to make that dream a possibility by keeping your options open. When one door closes, remember that there will always be another one if that particular door closes.

The problem that people have is that they give up at the first hurdle. Supposing you wanted to start a driving school because your passion is driving and you think you would be rather good at it. You then find that the area in which you live already has sufficient driving schools and that it would be unlikely to work. The man without positive attitude would simply give up on the idea and continue to live in his unsatisfactory life, putting the dream to one side. The man who is willing to keep his options open would look into other jobs in the area where he can employ his passion of driving and that may include totally different ideas to his original one, but ideas that are more viable. For example, he may find that there are jobs which pay sufficiently for driving cars at weddings, or he may be able to get a job as a driver which would expand his experience even more and allow him to use his passion as a way to get into something more viable later. Keeping your options open is essential if you want to find success. Those that close the door to potential success are usually those who are left with negative feelings once their initial idea doesn't work. It doesn't have to stop there. Keeping your options open means opening your mind to other possibilities.

I can cite an example here of a lady who wanted to become an ice skating star. Looking into it, she found that she had to go through all of the qualifiers and that her performance would have to be up to a certain level which she knew she could not attain without the help of a coach. The coach was out of the question because she didn't haÐČ.ve the financial resources to take on that coach. Instead, she looked at ways in which she could use skating as a potential career move, thus getting known in skating circles. That was a real possibility.

"I didn't know what I was going to do," she said, "but it had to involve skating. Then I noticed a very obscure advertisement at the bottom of a local newspaper and knew that it opened potential doors. It was for a skating instructor for kids. What I didn't realize at the time that I went for the job was that I would find more passion in teaching kids than I thought possible. Now instead of going forward into becoming a professional, I help others to take that ride of a lifetime and that's actually given me more joy than it would have done had I taken the choice to hire a coach and do it myself."

No matter how obscure your dream, you can realize it in some small way that leads you to where you should be. You may not know where that is at this moment in time but if you keep your options open and move in the way that fate allows you to, you may find that your dream is easier to realize than you first thought it would be.

Positive belief in your goals and positive belief in yourself opens up all of the avenues in life that are closed to negative people. The negative person dismisses the idea of doing anything other than the dream that they hold dear. They then feel disappointment and disillusionment when something stands between them and their dream and they don't look elsewhere for potential. When you switch mindset and go from positive to negative, you sabotage your own chances at happiness. If you try to explain that to some people, they can't get their heads around the fact that flexibility and optimism are essential and that negative instincts and thoughts will always block the path to their success.

Positivity fires up the imagination and allows you think "outside the box" so that your ideas don't seem so impossible. You can then work on your ideas and fit them into your life so that they work for everyone. In the above case scenario, the skater found that the work she was doing fitted with her lifestyle, caused no problems with her partner and did not take her away from home as much as being a professional skater would have.

That pleased her and it also pleased her partner and solved a lot of the issues that had been brewing up between them because of her partner's worry about his wife being away from home for long periods of time. There are solutions and there are ways that you can fit your career into your lifestyle without letting go of the passion and that's what she managed to do by keeping her options open.

CHAPTER FIVE

WHERE FEAR COMES INTO THE PICTURE

You may not be aware of it but many people fail to succeed because they are too afraid of failure and don't try. It seems easier to live a mundane life than to believe that you can succeed. Thus these are people whose lives will always be mundane. You need to find a way to get beyond this fear and learn that failure isn't really as bad as you are making it out to be. In fact, changing your view toward failure may help you to make it something that you no longer dread. People are conditioned to succeed. They are conditioned to taking the safe road. Thus, when you decide to take a road that is unfamiliar, you will feel genuine fear and will have to overcome it. Positive attitude helps you and if you can look at your fears in a much more rational way, you will see that these are just small things that can be overcome. The fear of rejection, the fear of failure and the fear of the unknown only stay as fears if you continue to feel rejected, continue to fail and don't learn about the unknown so that it becomes a more familiar and comfortable place.

Society today tends to encourage people to always stay on the safe road. We are told how important it is that we follow models given to us by those people whose lives seem to be conforming to society standards to such an extent that these are shown to us as examples of how we should be. However, if you are always afraid of rejection, chances are that you will hold yourself back. There are other ways to look at these negative situations to help you to maximize the benefit that you can glean from them.

STEP 20 – LEARNING HOW TO HANDLE REJECTION

Rejection is something that is going to happen during the course of your life. When it does, instead of fearing it, embrace it. What it means is that you need to change direction and you should use it as a lesson in self-development. It helps you to understand your strengths and your weaknesses and if you are ultimately to be happy in your life, this helps you considerably. When you tell a child that the child has something wrong, you don't do it to make the child feel bad. We see negative feedback as something that rejects the way that we are, but sometimes it can be so valuable and help us to grow as human beings. The way to gracefully handle rejection is not to be afraid of it. It is to thank the person who gives you feedback and use that feedback to move on in your life.

Rejection comes in all kinds of forms. For example, if you go for an interview for that ideal job and then get your application rejected, you may feel that it's the end of the world, when in fact, fate may have better things in store for you. Never see rejection as being the end of the road. It's the beginning of another road. A poet that I knew was extremely clever with words and yet when she received a rejection from a poetry contest, she was very shocked at what she learned. The poetry contest was based on the format of a sonnet. She truly believed that her poem was in sonnet format but there are several and it did not conform to the sonnet format that was specified. She had worked hard on the poems but she learned something valuable from the rejection and went on to becoming one of the most astute writers of sonnets in their correct format. The rejection was a positive move forward in her life and introduced something to her that she may otherwise never have been aware of.

Rejection doesn't mean there is something wrong with you. For example, if you are not given the dream job that you hoped for, it isn't a personal reflection on who you are so stop taking it so personally. Chances are that the employer had to interview many people for that job. All the rejection means is that someone else made a better impression. Learn from it. Analyze the way in which you handled the interview and decide what you could change if you had the opportunity of another one for a similar type of job. You learn from mistakes all of the time. If you look logically at a child who is learning to walk. He/she may fall over and cry. It hurts the pride but it also hurts to not be able to do something. If the child was to take the same attitude as many grown up people do at the sight of some kind of failure, he/she would not get up and try again. The child would simply accept that crawling is a safer way forward. Of course, it doesn't make sense but that's what those who cannot accept rejection restrict themselves to. They stop trying. Just like the child, you need to dust yourself off, tell yourself that it wasn't meant to be and look for other avenues, learning from your rejection and getting better at presenting yourself for the next. Positivity is what it's all about. In fact, those who have belief in themselves won't even flinch at the thought of rejection. They just see it as one door closing and a new one opening.

STEP 21 – LEARNING TO HANDLE FAILURE

Failure means such a negative thing to those that let it. Let's take a look at a situation and see how it can be turned around. You have painted a magnificent image and want to get it out to galleries where your work will be appreciated by others and you can gain a reputation as an artist.

"Your work is not what we are looking for at this time."

You can either feel like a failure or you can use it to develop your ability to please that particular market. Here's how. You can choose to submit the work to another market and take notes of what was rejected so that you can try something totally different for the first market that rejected you. You haven't failed. Start thinking of this in a different way. If you gain information, how can it be seen as a failure? You learned that the particular market you aimed for was not looking for what you sent them. Thus, it's a learning experience and that's something that is positive.

The other thing is that if you hang your paintings in an unsuitable gallery, you probably won't get the type of audience that you want, so the rejection makes you look into alternatives. Along the way, you may find that you see the possibility of selling prints which means that for a small outlay you can get your artwork out there and gaining in popularity. You can even take this further and advertise to work on commissions. One artist that I know started out by drawing pictures of flowers. She found that she had such an eye for detail that she was able to work on miniatures and became a member of the Royal Institute for Miniature Art. Knowing that this would not earn her a living, she carried on with commissions for people and diversified by applying for jobs for card making companies and jigsaw manufacturers and secured a contract which has continued to pay her good money for the past ten years.

She handled failure by using it as a learning tool and if you are able to do this, you learn to diversify and not to put all of your eggs in one basket. If another market comes up for illustration, she will gladly take this on – as she has done when opportunities arise. The book that she was asked to illustrate was a book showing all the different species of birds and although this took time, it added to her portfolio which in turn adds weight to her resume.

If you go through life looking for where you failed instead of where you can succeed by changing your approach, you will never find that balance. Every time that failure is perceived, look at it objectively and learn something from it so that it is no longer a negative thing. That way, you begin to see what you perceived as failures to be lessons. These lessons open doors to potential and it is this potential that you need to harness if you want to succeed. They are there for everyone, but only those who aim for them will achieve them. If you give up the first time that you experience a rejection, then perhaps you need to rethink your passion because it's obviously not powerful enough to make you want to learn and move on.

STEP 22 – LEARNING EMPATHY

If people disappoint you with their perceptions of your success, it is easy to let this make you feel like you have failed. However, when you learn empathy, you are able to put yourself into their shoes and see a bigger picture instead of a narrower one. Many big business people do this by practicing Neuro Linguistic programming because it helps them to have a wider view. People with a wider view are more likely to succeed. When something happens that you see as negative, step back from it and think in the following way:

- What was the feedback I was given that made me feel negative?

- Why would that particular person feel like that? What fueled their thoughts?

- How can I change the approach so that it's acceptable to me as well as to others?

You need to address your fears and this allows you to do so with a positive mindset instead of automatically thinking that you did something wrong. Creativity and the sense of achievement is never lost if you can turn failure around and make it into a learning process. Supposing you want to be a clothes designer and are rejected from a company based on the fact that your portfolio doesn't match up to their requirements. Seeing the bigger picture, you have to understand that there are many markets within the fashion industry that cater for many different kinds of people. If you understand and can empathize with people, you will also gain a greater understanding of market needs and can offer your services in a position which suits your style because it does exist. It's just a question of understanding the market.

Empathy is valuable to relationships. It forges friendships because you also learn to listen to others and sometimes the greatest lessons that you can learn in life are those which you obtain through active listening. If you have a lot of positive friendships, these act as a barrier against being hurt because you always have their support and that's important when you are trying to discover who you are or what your dream is. People with no support from others feel alone and isolated, while people with empathy and lots of friends find it easy to pick up the pieces after what could be perceived as a failure and start again with the same level of optimism that they had before.

Thus mix with people and make them an important part of your life because everyone you know adds a rich dimension to your life that helps you to see more possibilities. This doesn't mean that you use people. It means that you listen and empathize and cultivate good solid friendships that will help you through times that are lean and that you will always help in the same way. Your happiness level depends upon having people that you can rely upon and that also respect you and the way that you are because this gives you confidence to try again.

STEP 23 – RECOGNIZE YOUR OWN WEAKNESSES

If you are aware that you have weaknesses, try all that you can to strengthen them or to find the kind of work where those weaknesses do not matter. When you persist in being involved in things that you know are your weak points, you are always going to feel weak. There are all kinds of interests in life and if you can recognize your weaknesses and work on them this helps you to feel less fearful of life. Don't be hard on yourself. You cannot know everything. All you can do is be the best person you can be.

The kind of weaknesses that I have in mind that will help you are:

- Your attitude toward life

- Your emotional instability

- Your dependence upon others

- Your inability to make friends

- Your mistrust in life

- Your inability to be flexible

There is only one person in the world that knows you through and through. Often, we get bad feedback from people but it may not necessarily be honest or even true. What you know about yourself is therefore of paramount importance to your happiness levels. If you know that you have a fault, then a little concentration on that area will always help you to develop your character so that you overcome that fault. The problem with negative faults is that they get in the way of dreams being realized. For example, if your emotional state depends upon you being in a relationship, that's not a good reason to be in a relationship. You have to learn to be happy as an individual without leaning on others to provide that happiness for you. If your attitude toward life is such that you sabotage your own chances of success, dissect it and find out what you do that stops you from succeeding. Alter your behavior or approach and see if this improves the quality of your life. You may find that it's your lack of positivity that is sabotaging all of your ideas and if that is the case, you need to get back on track, envision those dreams and keep heading for them regardless of setbacks.

You have to understand that every change must be one that moves toward being positive because it is positive attitude that is going to be your ally through all the changes in your life. Positivity is what you are aiming at achieving.

CHAPTER SIX

STEPS TO GAINING CONFIDENCE IN YOURSELF

If you feel confident about who you are, then you don't doubt your own authenticity. You are able to go forward in your life knowing that you have the power to make things happen. In this world, people do not look after themselves as they should. It's a competitive world, but you do need to respect your need for reflection, time sleeping and keeping your body in tip top condition. This helps you to feel much better about yourself and also allows the mind sufficient time to heal during the sleep process. The REM stage of sleep is essential to all who want to be at their most productive. There are other ways as well in which you can maximize your own potential. Let me explain a little about how the body works. Just as when you injure yourself, sleep helps to mend the injury, sleep also helps to mend the mind. You need that sleep to get your life back in balance. The hormones that are released during sleep are the same ones that make you wake up in the morning feeling refreshed. Your mind will work more efficiently when you are able to respect its need for sleep. You also need to have time to yourself and increase your learning skills because this helps you to have a constant stream of new ideas.

STEP 24 – TAKE SOME "ME" TIME

The reason that you need this is that it is a time for you to refresh your thoughts and to feel good about your life. If you deprive yourself of "me" time, you can get to a point where you feel resentful of those around you. That doesn't help your positivity levels. One way in which you could do this is to opt for the exercise of having time to yourself every day and learning meditation. I would suggest that you take this up with a teacher so that you have the impetus to follow it through, but this strengthens the mind and makes you much more aware of your own thoughts and wishes. You may also want to take up a sport or do something that is creative. This "me" time for an adult is like play time for a child. Without any playtime, a childhood is incomplete and the creative part of the child is neglected. It's much the same with adults and you need to allow yourself that time. You may want to go swimming, discover a new kind of food or you may simply want to switch off, go to the park with a good book and read. Whatever floats your boat, you need to make time for it.

Why "me" time is important

"Me" time re-establishes the fact that you are an individual and that you have a right to do the things that you want to do. If you are deprived of this, you can feel enclosed or stifled and can begin to experience negative emotions such as resentment. Imagine the new mom who is stuck at home every day and does not get adult conversation. She may have had a very good job where she had social contact every day. However nice it is to have a new baby, she craves that company but cannot have it because there is no one to help her or to take the load from her.

In a case like this, paying a very good babysitter for a couple of hours so that she can get out and do her own thing will take away much of the resentment and negativity that she feels. Perhaps parents can help out or perhaps there is a friend that she can swap favors with so that she doesn't lose that part of herself that she feels is important to her.

Being a new mom isn't the only time that people lose "me" time. A man may feel that he is under an obligation to work 6 days a week and then feels pressure on his day off to do all of the chores he has no other time to do. That means, in effect, that he is working seven days a week and getting no real "me" time. No wonder he builds up resentment. In a case such as this, he would need to organize things so that he can do a few of the spare jobs in the early evening and free up the weekend so that at least one day a week, he can do the things that he wants to do. There has to be a work/home life balance and when this is missing, it's easy for negativity to set in.

If you are in a relationship and want that "me" time, it's important to discuss this with your partner in a rational and non-accusatory way. If your partner knows about your discontent, two heads can often come up with solutions faster than one. However, you should never lay it onto your partner as a negative thing. Let your partner know how much this means to you and tell him/her that you would be a lot happier if you had this little bit of time to do something that you really want to do. Keep everything positive and never include any criticism or negativity in your talks because this just achieves a bad atmosphere and very little resolution.

STEP 25 – TAKE UP NEW THINGS

It's a good idea to keep your mind open to new ideas. This is what feeds the most successful of people. They don't just stick to one thing. They diversify. That's what keeps them fired up and enthused with new ideas. It is these new ideas that make the difference between a dream lasting and a dream dying. If you don't have new things in your life, all your influences can become stale. You need to read up on new ideas, follow them through and feel positive toward all the changes that you see happening around you. There is an expression which is very relevant. "Go with the flow!" I was offered a chance to take up a cooking course recently and cooking is something that gives me very little pleasure indeed. I laughed at the idea initially, but when I looked further into it, what I was gaining was worth trying something new. The chef who was French was actually willing to impart information where I would learn to make delicious treats for people for Christmas, so instead of turning up my nose at the chance, I gained from it and can now spread that joy among my friends which gives them and me more pleasure than I would have thought possible. There are always new ideas around the corner and one of them may just lead you to the creation of a new dream. The potential that people miss out on because they are not prepared to try something new is wasted opportunity waiting for everyone. Some choices will not be as fruitful, but they are useful because if you don't enjoy these pastimes that means that you have a narrower field in which to search for your dream existence, so it's helpful to know that.

STEP 26 – BELIEVE IN YOURSELF

No matter who doubts you, as long as you have belief in yourself, that's enough. Don't let yourself feed from other people's negativity. If you can keep yourself motivated and keep your own faith in what you are doing, then that should be enough. You will find that if you are able to incorporate meditation into your life that you will see things differently. It isn't about what other people think of you. It's about how you live with yourself and your belief system. You are all that you have. Outside opinions shouldn't sway you because that's all they are – opinions. You need to keep on track and believe in your dream because it's that belief that fires up your enthusiasm to carry on.

So how do you learn to believe in yourself? Making affirmations about the things that you want to be included in your life is helpful because they give you a dream to believe in. Not being afraid of change will help you as well because every time you go through a new situation and come out of the other side of it equally positive, you re-affirm your own ability to take life in a flexible manner. If you learn to take rejection in your stride and learn from it, you begin to believe in your own ability to accept things and to move beyond them. If you have little confidence in yourself, you need to work through the earlier stages of this book and try to find the things that really do fulfill your dreams and work toward them. These help you to have purpose in life. People seek purpose and when there is no purpose, it's very hard to believe in yourself. Thus, establish a purpose, establish a dream and work toward it, knowing yourself sufficiently well to know that whatever door opens in front of you, you are ready to take the challenge.

STEP 27 – READ AND LEARN

I once got told that I would never live overseas. It had always been my dream. People didn't think that I would be able to survive a life without deep conversation and let's face it, my skills in language were not that great. However, my dream was bigger than that and that's what most people failed to see. Because I believed in the dream, I taught myself the language and am fluent now. Read and learn because when you stop learning, you also stop your dreams in their tracks. Don't be too stubborn to learn. Learning is positive reinforcement and helps you to become more confident and able to live your dream. In my particular case, I was not only able to converse, but I learned the intricacies of the language and there doesn't come a point when you stop learning as there will always be something else you can add to your list of achievements. If you fail at one thing, try another. You don't have to be the world's greatest intellect to gain something from learning and perhaps rather than academic skills, you may find that you prefer manual skills because not everyone sees learning in the same light.

If there are areas in your life where you feel that you need to strengthen your ability, then do it. You gain so much from lessons which help you to live your dream. If you can't speak in public, take a course that will help you. If you fear moving on in a new direction, learn all about it so that you don't have stumbling blocks getting in your way. Imagine wanting to learn pottery. The first time that you throw the clay, you are not going to create the perfect pot, but by watching others and learning, you gain confidence in that given craft and you also learn to produce things of your own from your own ideas. There is so much scope for learning.

By learning about things, you help yourself to gain even more confidence and that's when magic starts to happen. You have to look at every aspect of your life that is negative and ask yourself why. Then you need to firm up your knowledge so that those areas of doubt become areas of certainly. Knowledge is exceedingly powerful and when you gain it, you know that you are going the right way. Remember the first time that you rode a bike on your own without your dad supporting it? I remember that as if it was yesterday and it's a good job that I do. That's the same feeling that I get every time I achieve something new through my own learning skills. It's a wonderful feeling and fires up enthusiasm like nothing else that I know. If I ever find a question in life that I can't answer, I follow it up with a search for information and with the Internet everyone is capable of doing that. The amount of learning power that people have these days is no different, but the source of information is so vast that we no longer have the excuse of not knowing about something. Use your spare time to answer all of your questions and enjoy the journey.

CHAPTER SEVEN

YOUR INTERACTIONS WITH OTHERS

Did you know that every time you do something positive, with no strings attached, you gain more confidence in who you are? It's true. In many books, you will find that volunteerism is used to help people with self-esteem issues. It is something that you can add to your life to help you to see your own value. You only see it if you can give without expecting anything in return. It humbles you, but it also shows you that you have a good heart and that's important on the road to success. So how does volunteerism work to help you to feel happier about your life? If you really can give without expectations, you gain a better insight into what giving is all about. Imagine a woman who gives her child a first rate education but expects something in return.

What will inevitably happen is that the child will feel obliged to live up to those expectations or the woman will feel disappointed because the child didn't. Laying that trip on a child is pretty awful but some people who give are like that. They don't actually volunteer anything if there is some kind of reward expected. Volunteerism in the truest sense is giving something with absolutely no expectations of anything and that's when you start to feel good about yourself. You don't need someone else to validate who you are any more. You already know and that's much more valuable than any of your expectations of others can be.

In this world, people are self-reliant. They need to be complete in and of themselves rather than needing the perpetual validation of others. When people with self esteem are asked to volunteer it is because this gives them a sense of value without actually putting any strings upon what it is that they give. A woman working in a homeless dog shelter will derive much pleasure from working with animals because she is doing a useful job that no one else wants to do. She doesn't expect anything of the animals at all, but she will gain such wonderful encouragement from seeing the dogs thrive. This translates into helping her to address her self-esteem issues.

STEP 28 – GIVE SOMETHING OF YOU TO SOMEONE ELSE

In this case, this exercise will help you to feel positive. Bake a cake for a neighbor, cookies for the local school fete or simply help out in a soup kitchen. Don't do it for the reward. Don't stand around waiting for everyone to recognize how good you are because that's not what it's about. Give and then walk away knowing that you did so without the need for other people to validate what you did. This self-validation is all it takes to help you to stay positive. Know the difference between volunteering and making yourself out to be a martyr and don't fall for giving to such an extent that you deprive yourself of valuable time in your life. People who do this tend to become negative and feel that the world owes them something. In fact, give with a good heart or not at all because if you give with anything less, you won't gain the positive benefits that you would otherwise reap.

STEP 29 – TELEPHONE SOMEONE WHO CARES

We all get out of line in our lives and have regrets. Sometimes a friend deserves a little more attention than we have given them. When you telephone someone, forget about talking about you and concentrate on listening to that friend. The reason I say this is that it teaches you that the world doesn't revolve around you alone. Sometimes, you need to open your ears to listening and becoming a good listener is very valuable on the road to success. You don't even need a reason. Just phone someone who makes you feel good and make them feel good for a while. Positive vibes do wonders.

Take the opportunity to ask their news. Let them know that you miss them but make the call about them, rather than about you. You must have experienced people who telephone you to tell you all of their good fortune. People do this all of the time. The difference here is that you are not doing that. You are phoning up to show someone else that you care about his/her life – rather than bragging about yours. When you get into the habit of phoning friends with no motive other than to see how they are, this fills your life with a lot of positivity. People are more attracted to you as a person and it's more likely that you will be able to distinguish between those friends who are genuine and those who are not.

Active listening means not interrupting their chain of speech. Listen and encourage them to talk. Behind the words that they are saying, you may find that you can get to know people so well that you know when a visit is needed and this may just make someone you know very happy indeed. By reaching out to people and then letting them into your life, you retain good friendships and these contribute positivity to your life. Even if you haven't phoned them for a long time, making the effort breaks the ice between you and fosters good long term friendships. Active listening also allows you to get to know people better and when you do, you can decide if they add positivity to your life or if they are looking for one sided relationships. Stick to those friendships where give and take is in equal measures as these relationships will pass the test of time.

STEP 30 – DISCUSS YOUR DREAMS WITH SOMEONE WHO MATTERS

Often we have dreams and we don't discuss them with the people who matter. The problem with this kind of thinking is that it does nothing to firm up that dream. If you want something badly enough in your life, make it a part of your everyday life so that it isn't just you working toward it. You need to have family and friends on your side and if they don't know what that dream is, how can you expect them to understand? We often go through life thinking that communicating our dreams isn't important, but it is. When other people are involved, you are given new ideas and even if you don't use all of them, chances are that some will add to your idea and make it more viable. You can have anything that you want in this life, but you need to have people that matter to you on your side or at least ready, willing and able to feed you positivity during the time that you need to make that dream a reality.

Jennifer and her husband talked about her love of horses. Living in the city, there was not much chance for her to follow through on her dreams, but her husband was open to the possibility of moving to the country. He was a qualified doctor and wanted to specialize in working with handicapped children. He suggested that they learn more about the work that people do with kids like this that involves horses. While they were investigating, Jennifer discovered that she had a natural knack for working with kids and combining her love for horses. With the right kind of training, she was able to team up with her husband and open a center for the handicapped where they both got to live what they saw as their dreams. Now imagine the case scenario had Jennifer never mentioned her secret passion. Her dream would never have been realized and it was only by discussing it with her husband that they were able to put A and B together to make C.

The other thing about discussing your dream is that people who care about you may be able to come up with options that work to help you to realize your dreams. Choose someone that you trust and if they do not show the same level of enthusiasm as you, then don't be put off by it. At least they will know why you take the different turns on the road that lead you to realizing that dream.

STEP 31 – THE KEY IS ALWAYS GOING TO BE COMMUNICATION

Communication counts for everything. If you are able to explain ideas and ideals to others and convince them, then you are well on your way to success. However, what if people fail to see your dream as viable? What do you do then? If you can communicate with others, you can feed off their positivity and come up with fresh ideas that will work for you. Communication is a two way thing. Listen and learn. Speak and voice your opinions, but never criticize others. Every time that you do, you may just be squashing someone else's dream. Learn that relationships and friendships are a two way thing and that if you need positivity from people, you must also give positivity.

The people that you surround yourself with are paramount to your success in life. Treat others as you wish to be treated and let their positivity help you through times that are negative. Let yours shine when they need it to. It's very much a communication issue and those who succeed are those that feel true empathy as well as wishing to fulfill their own dreams. You can never fulfill your dreams at the expense of others, or it will indeed be a hollow victory and one that will not have lasting happiness attached to it. You can't gain success from trampling over others. You can gain it by wishing them well, even if their ideas do not gel with yours. Be kind to people around you. Understand that your dreams are not the same as theirs but that theirs require just as much respect from you as you expect respect from them.

Happiness and fulfillment come from working through ideas in a very positive manner, rather than loading others with different views with negativity. You need positive feedback and you also need to give it. It may be someone else's dream that you are discussing, but it feels good if you are able to help them to realize that dream. This is a lesson that parents should learn as well, as many parents try to stifle the creativity of their children for all of the wrong reasons. If you child told you that he wanted to be an artist, you would probably think that there's not much chance of that, especially when being an artist doesn't fall in with your ideas of a good career move. That child may just have talent. Parents have this stereotype image of what children should do with their lives and sometimes need to step outside of their comfort zones and support and encourage the child whose ideas are different. By communicating in an open way, you are able to gage how viable that dream is rather than just dismissing it because it doesn't fall in with your ideas and ideals.

It's the same with your ideas. If you need to discuss these with friends and family, get all of your information ready and present them with concrete ideas that they can help you to build on. Positive reinforcement comes from positive conversation. Communication is very important indeed when you are trying to live your life in positive mode.

CHAPTER EIGHT

THINGS YOU NEED TO QUIT

In this section, we deal with the keys that are stopping you from succeeding. You need to be aware of these as they may be standing in the way of your own positivity and of your ultimate success. If you heed to warning given by these points, you will find that you learn to be more positive in your life because you are not laying the path to failure. Remember, a failure is a failure – no matter how small it is – and adds to your feeling of never being able to reach your goal. Yes, we have asked you to change your view about the way that you see failure, but it's a hard task to do and will take time to accomplish. In the meantime, here are the top things you need to quit if you want to be happy and successful. Positive thinking will help you along the way.

STEP 33 – STOP MAKING FALSE PROMISES TO YOURSELF AND OTHERS

If you are one of those people who start things with all good intentions and then stop mid-stream, you need to work out a different way to handle the things you have to do. Your system isn't working. You may have come across people that make promises and never keep them and when you start things you won't finish, you are doing the same thing. For example, people who start diets and don't follow them through are typical. People who say they will give up smoking and then fail are another example. You need to do things with all of your heart knowing that you will finish whatever it was that you started. If you set yourself up with goals that you know you cannot reach you are sabotaging your chances of success in life because you will always be disappointed that you didn't make it to the finish line.

If you want to know how to step off that bandwagon, then the answer lies in the goals that you set for yourself. Make them achievable. Start off with small goals so that those around you can regain confidence in the fact that you will keep your promise and do the things you say you will. These goals should be things that you know you can see through to the end. Remember, each time that you do this, you build up positive reinforcement that you are someone of your word and people will begin to trust you more. If you always say you will do things but never do them, that doesn't help your reputation. It is better to have a small goal and celebrate your victory than to be surrounded by people whose only opinion of you is based upon your personal failures.

STEP 34 – STOP PUTTING THINGS OFF FOR ANOTHER DAY

That day may never come. Have you ever seen the vicious circle that happens when someone has a payday loan? They borrow money from next months' pay packet and then have to pay it back, leaving them short again the following month. When you put things off, you eat into the time that you tomorrow. Thus you reach tomorrow already in debt and thus this stops you from having the time that you need to achieve your goals. If you can't do something, try asking for help or getting someone else to do it. If you carry on putting things off until tomorrow, you fill your future with obligations that get in the way of reaching out beyond your normal limits to grab that dream.

Write down what you are going to achieve tomorrow and keep to it. This may be small things at first, but that's the way the psych works. When you achieve one thing, it drives you onward to achieve something else. My deeds for today, for example are to sweep up the leaves in the garden and clean the windows. They are doable and at the end of the day I will have the satisfaction that these jobs have been done and won't need to be done again for a while. I could have added all the housework, cleaning the car and going into town for shopping, but that's not the way it works. It's not how many things you achieve, it's about starting something and actually finishing it. Celebrate the end of the job. Show the world and your conscience your own capability by being positive and positively reinforcing the fact that when you say you will do something, you actually will.

STEP 35 – TAKE RESPONSIBILITY AND STOP BLAMING

When you blame someone or something for not being able to do a task that you were supposed to do, you are telling the whole world it wasn't your fault. You may not know it but you are making yourself a victim and people don't like victims very much. They are surrounded by negative vibes and are always the ones who have all the misfortunes of the world cast upon them. In fact, it's become so corny that people also avoid victims because these are people who don't take responsibility or ownership of their own destiny. "It wasn't my fault the relationship finished." This may be something that you hear all of the time, but in fact if a relationship finishes, it's the fault of two people. It's just that those who say this are not ready to accept any responsibility. "I couldn't make the deadline because my kids tore up my paperwork." It sounds like a viable excuse but then if you delve further – why did the kids have access to the paperwork in the first place? The fact is that the buck stops with you. Take responsibility for errors because when you do, you can learn from them and move forward in a much more positive way without causing waves that make other people's lives miserable.

If you do make errors along the way, forgive yourself for them and learn by them. It's no big deal. However, it becomes a big deal when you don't acknowledge your part in the failure and blame others for it. "It was their fault for making so much noise" becomes "It was my fault for trying to work in a noisy environment. Next time I will remove myself to a quieter room." There are always going to be two ways of looking at things and it's important that you realize that changing your viewpoint and taking blame out of the picture makes it easier for you to achieve your goal the next time around.

STEP 36 – LEAVE YOUR EXPECTATIONS BEHIND

I have a favorite quotation that I use all of the time. "Blessed is he who expects nothing, for he shall never be disappointed." I am not sure who said it but it's very relevant. Think of a parent who gives a child a private education expecting that child to go into the legal profession. The child grows up and wants to follow his heart in photography. Thus, the parent's expectations are thwarted and they feel bitterly disappointed. If you don't expect anything, everything that you do get becomes even more positive. You get a letter of thanks that you were not expecting and it makes everything you have done worthwhile. You get a telephone call out of the blue offering you a new job simply because your character is the right kind of character for that job. You didn't expect it and when it comes, it builds up your confidence. Expectations are confidence busters. They break you into little pieces. Instead of having expectations, go through life having a reality because that's more tangible and less likely to make you feel disappointed.

It is good to have ambitions and you may see ambitions as being expectations, but they are not exactly on a par with expectations. Your ambition may be to become a concert pianist. However, you know that it takes a lot of work to get there. You set little targets along the way that take you one or two steps further along the road toward your ambition. You don't expect to be a concert pianist without all the effort it takes to get you there.

Drop the expectations. Take the practical steps that lead you to being what you want to be, rather than being perpetually disappointed by your own inappropriate expectations.

STEP 37 – STOP BEING A DOORMAT

You may not immediately understand what is meant by that but if you are the type of person who says "yes" when you mean "no" or would rather say "no" you are well on your way to becoming a doormat. You put off your dreams in favor of the wishes of others. You do things that go far and beyond friendship just because you lack confidence and think that it will give you a little "street credibility." Well, I have news for you. It doesn't make you popular and it doesn't help your confidence in the slightest bit. In fact, you are likely to end up feeling badly used and miserable. You have to get beyond this. If someone has asked you to do something that you really do not want to do, you need to learn to say "no."

The trouble is that people think that if they say "no" they won't be liked any more. It's time for a reality check. Look at people who you really admire or love and watch how they do it. They know when it's the right time to say "no" and they don't let people walk all over them, but they still get respect from people. How do they do it? They simply know their own limitations and they have set boundaries which tell them what is acceptable and what is not. They gain respect from others because of those boundaries. They are friendly and cheerful because they don't allow themselves to be someone's doormat. The moment that you become someone that others can wipe their feet on, you lose their respect and your own self-esteem. If you want to work toward your dreams, you need to stop being this person that does things he/she doesn't want to do. Learn to say "no."

These are the biggest hurdles toward moving in on your dream. You will find that each one of these is something you need to work on for a specific purpose. If you do not work on them, the chances of your dreams being fulfilled is hampered. When you do work on them, you learn a sense of inner peace that helps you to concentrate on what's important to you and gain respect along the way.

The best thing that I ever did in my life was to quit a job that made me feel like a second class citizen. It paid well, but it didn't pay enough to compensate for the way that I felt every night when I went home to bed. I took on another job that didn't pay as well, and where people treated me with respect. It wasn't a high profile job like the other one, but what I learned is that other people's idea of high profile and my own definition were different. High profile to me means something that makes me feel great and gives me all of the exposure that I need to be successful. It didn't take a Calvin Kline suit to get me there once I understood that this superficial nonsense was what was making my life a misery.

Reach for your dreams. Know what they are and if any of the pointers in this chapter sound like something that you would do, find a way to stop because it's essential that you do. Your happiness, confidence levels and your level of positivity depend upon it.

CONCLUSION

This book has covered a lot of ground. Positive attitude really feeds success and if you go through the keys that have been mentioned, you can fulfill your dreams. Some will be easier than others. Some will seem impossible, although everything that I have suggested within the pages of this book is possible. Positivity is something that surrounds you when you are on the road to success. It spurs you on. It keeps you enthused and on track. It also makes you feel great about your life. Since the course of your lifetime is only going to be a span of 100 years, that doesn't give you a lot of time to chase dreams. 20 years of that may be dedicated to growing up and schooling. That leaves you eighty years. Then, you are going to have to take off all of the time spent working – that is of course unless you can add your work to your dream.

In the book I have tried to give ideas in a very clear way because I know people who have self-esteem issues and find it hard to be positive. When I explained the simplicity of chasing your dreams to them, they were able to grasp the concept in a better way than had I explained the concept in convoluted complexity. Yes, all of this can be proven by science, by certain religious practices and even medically. If you feed the brain with positivity, you get positive results. Positive results lead to success stories. If you then add the elements of validation, affirmation (which is self-validation) and great results, what ensues is something almost magical. You achieve what you once thought was impossible.

Surrounding yourself with positive vibes helps you to pick up on those vibes and become positive in your own right. Meditation helps you to focus that positivity and even if you never become the best at performing yoga, it helps you to feel even more positive. Then you have the aspect of creativity. Keep this channel alive and you spark off new ideas which add to your dream and help you to realize it. The negative aspects of life are those which will destroy your dreams if you let them. We have talked about how people become their own worst enemy by insisting upon being victims. Somehow, people with low self-esteem feel that becoming a victim is the only way to get noticed. The problem behind that flawed way of thinking is that you get noticed for all of the wrong things. You become a drama queen and people laugh at you. Thus, when they do, you lose more self-esteem and do not gain any happiness from it at all.

If you read the chapter on things you need to avoid, you may find that you have been sabotaging your own potential to succeed and can start to make your way into stopping behaviors that feed negative results. I was once surrounded by people who thought that I should do certain things within my life and to a degree, I went along with it. Then, in middle age, I suddenly realized that I only had a limited number of years left in my life. That wasn't a drama queen moment. It was a reality. Because I had been so busy living other people's idea of who I should be, I had lost the one core thing that could have made me happy. Somewhere amidst the chaos of my life, I had lost who I was. When you get to the stage that you are no longer pleasing yourself and your life is not one that suits you, you do need to address this with positive thinking and innovation. In my particular case, quitting the job that was killing my own personality was the first step.

Then I decided to remove all negative influences from my life. That wasn't as straightforward as it may seem since some people are very clever at hiding their negative vibes but if you are always doing things for people without really wanting to, then you need to recognize why and move away from becoming a doormat.

I listened to a life coach about achievement. If you want to achieve a great salary, you can and there is nothing stopping you except the limitations YOU place on yourself. If you want to live in the country, stop making that city workplace the reason for stopping yourself from actually enjoying life. If you can't commute, you can always take up a career that takes you in a different and happier direction. You don't have to be this person that people put a label on.

Positive thinking changes everything. Your life becomes happier. Your friendships become more developed. Your career takes a new direction. You may even find yourself doing something you have always wanted to do, but have put to the back of your mind simply because you never thought it was possible. What stopped you all these years was your own negativity toward the idea. Stop limiting yourself. There are few limitations in life and those that are there are usually because YOU put them there.

The dream is something that we can all grasp. The earlier you grasp it, the less resentment you have about the years that have passed that were not happy. Driven by positivity, find out who you are. Take the journey of discovery and find out what your true roots are. Meditation can help you to discover this, but if you cannot meditate or concentrate for that long, try this. Close your eyes and imagine a perfect world. It will be different for everyone. Imagine the people within that world. Imagine the type of home in which you will be living. Imagine the country in which this dream takes place. See it all in color and use your own visualization to help you to achieve that which you see as the ideal.

When you have definite thoughts about what your dream is, that gives you something to aim toward. Remember, when bad things happen, these are merely changes in direction. Don't see them as anything more than this. Learn from them. Be with positive people and share your dream. Let it gradually become your reality. It can and does happen, and the visualization of the dream may be something that you can step back into whenever you have doubts in yourself or the way in which your life is going. Sit in a comfortable chair, close your eyes and see the dream. If you can see it clearly enough, it cannot escape. Nor can you escape the fate that will take you there. Positive belief in your dream, in yourself and in the people around you will help you on the way to fulfilling everything you ever wanted to. As you get toward the dream, flesh it out with more detail. Always have something to aim at because part of being human is having positive input all of the time and that includes ambition and hope. Once you achieve that, you will understand how simple the recipe for life is and how attainable. Then you will see that positivity toward others will also help them to achieve their hopes and dreams.

FREE BONUS GUIDE: "5 BEST SECRETS TO ELIMINATING STRESS AND WORRY"

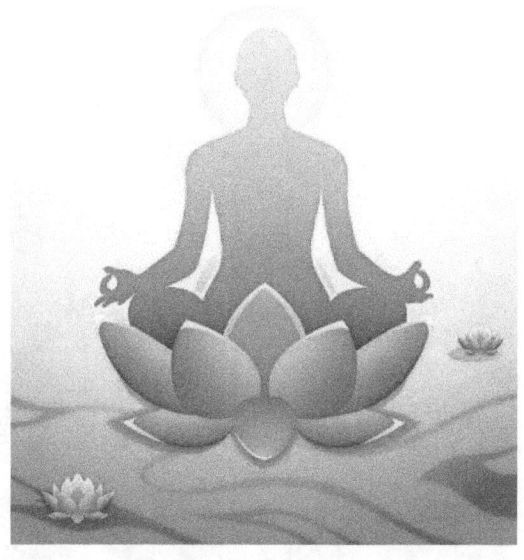

FREE BONUS "CLAIM YOUR GUIDE"

BELOW FOR YOUR BONUS

HTTPS://SUCCESS321.LEADPAGES.CO/FREEBODYMINDSOUL/